STAY SLIM

Chattram Trivedi

PREFACE

The book is guiding you with small tricks to manage your body weight , diet and food in a simple form.

STAY SLIM

(Book of Tricks to stay fit)

Chattram Trivedi

NUTRITION TIPS

1. Eat smaller portions.

2. Focus on whole, unprocessed foods.

3. Eat slowly and chew thoroughly.

4. Avoid sugary drinks.

5. Drink water before meals.

6. Add more fiber to your diet.

7. Include protein in every meal.

8. Use smaller plates for meals.

9. Avoid eating straight from packages.

10. Limit added sugars and artificial sweeteners.

11. Choose healthy fats like olive oil and avocados.

12. Cook meals at home.

13. Avoid late-night snacking.

14. Plan meals ahead of time.

15. Start meals with a salad or broth-based soup.

16. Snack on raw veggies or nuts.

17. Reduce salt intake to prevent bloating.

18. Add spices to flavor food instead of sauces.

19. Limit alcohol consumption.

20. Avoid skipping breakfast.

HYDRATION HABITS

21. Drink at least 8 glasses of water daily.

22. Replace sodas with herbal teas.

23. Keep a water bottle with you at all times.

24. Infuse water with lemon, cucumber, or mint for flavor.

25. Drink green tea to boost metabolism.

Physical Activity Tips

26. Take the stairs instead of the elevator.

27. Walk for at least 30 minutes daily.

28. Stretch every morning.

29. Incorporate strength training exercises.

30. Do yoga to improve flexibility and balance.

31. Park farther away from entrances.

32. Try dancing as a workout.

33. Play with your kids or pets to stay active.

34. Use a standing desk when possible.

35. Walk or bike instead of driving.

36. Take regular breaks to move around.

37. Clean your house for extra movement.

38. Join a group exercise class for motivation.

39. Explore outdoor activities like hiking.

40. Use resistance bands for quick workouts.

MINDSET AND MENTAL HEALTH

41. Practice mindful eating.

42. Focus on progress, not perfection.

43. Avoid comparing yourself to others.

44. Set small, achievable goals.

45. Meditate daily to reduce stress.

46. Celebrate non-scale victories.

47. Stay positive and self-compassionate.

48. Keep a journal of your journey.

49. Avoid emotional eating by addressing triggers.

50. Visualize your long-term success.

SLEEP AND REST

51. Get 7-8 hours of sleep per night.

52. Stick to a consistent sleep schedule.

53. Avoid screens an hour before bedtime.

54. Create a calming bedtime routine.

55. Keep your bedroom cool and dark.

56. Avoid heavy meals before bed.

57. Reduce caffeine in the afternoon.

MEAL TIMING AND STRUCTURE

58. Eat at regular intervals.

59. Don't skip meals to avoid overeating later.

60. Stop eating when you're 80% full.

61. Practice intermittent fasting if it suits you.

62. Start the day with a protein-rich breakfast.

63. Have dinner at least 3 hours before bed.

Smart Grocery Shopping

64. Make a shopping list and stick to it.

65. Shop the perimeter of the store (fresh produce, protein).

66. Avoid shopping when hungry.

67. Read food labels carefully.

68. Choose fresh over processed foods.

Social Strategies

69. Share meals at restaurants.

70. Politely decline second helpings.

71. Surround yourself with health-conscious friends.

72. Choose active outings with friends.

73. Bring healthy dishes to gatherings.

HABITS AND LIFESTYLE

74. Meal prep to avoid unhealthy choices.

75. Keep healthy snacks on hand.

76. Avoid eating in front of the TV.

77. Keep tempting foods out of sight.

78. Use apps to track food and activity.

79. Reward yourself with non-food treats.

80. Focus on long-term habits, not diets.

NATURAL WEIGHT LOSS BOOSTERS

81. Add apple cider vinegar to meals.

82. Eat more probiotic-rich foods (yogurt, kimchi).

83. Avoid processed carbs like white bread.

84. Add cinnamon to stabilize blood sugar.

85. Eat dark chocolate in moderation to curb cravings.

86. Include green leafy vegetables in every meal.

87. Use lemon juice to reduce fat absorption.

88. Avoid fried foods; bake or steam instead.

89. Eat seasonal fruits and vegetables.

90. Choose whole grains like quinoa and oats.

STAYING CONSISTENT

91. Track your progress weekly.

92. Find an accountability partner.

93. Celebrate small milestones.

94. Adjust strategies when needed.

95. Be patient—results take time.

96. Focus on how you feel, not just weight.

97. Stay curious about new, healthy habits.

98. Avoid all-or-nothing thinking.

99. Embrace flexibility in your routine.

Remember: health is a lifelong journey and make your own plan to achieve it.

YOUR PLAN

KEY NOTES

KEY NOTES